GALVESTON DIET COOKBOOK

Comprehensive Guide to Easy, Delicious and Mouth-watering recipes for healthier lifestyles

BY

Mildred Kent

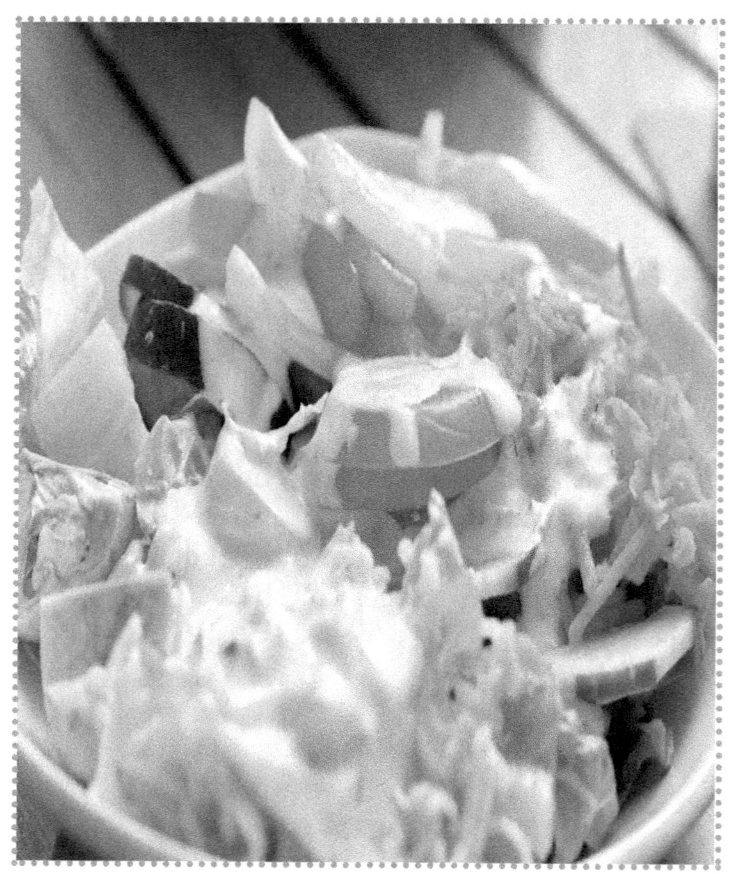

TABLE OF CONTENT

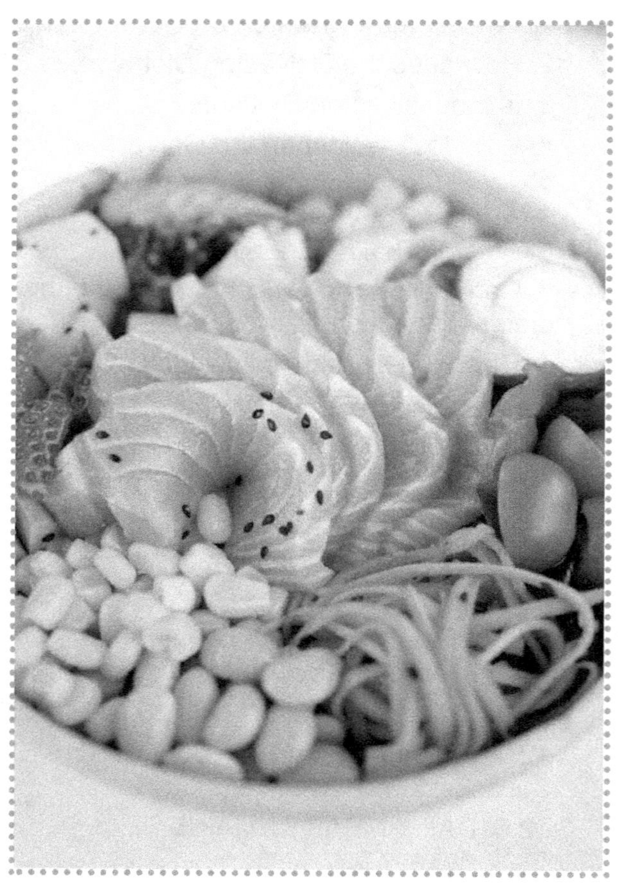

CHAPTER ONE

1. Introduction to the Galveston Diet

Welcome to the world of the Galveston Diet, a revolutionary approach to wellness and weight management that's gaining traction for its effectiveness and simplicity. In this introduction, we'll explore into the core philosophy and principles of the Galveston Diet, exploring its origins, development, and the science behind it.

1.2 Overview of the Galveston Diet philosophy and principles

The Galveston Diet is founded on the principle of balancing hormones to promote sustainable weight loss and overall health. Unlike many fad diets that focus solely on calorie restriction or eliminating entire food groups, the Galveston Diet recognizes the importance of hormonal balance in regulating metabolism, appetite, and energy levels.

At the heart of the Galveston Diet philosophy are three key principles:

1. **Hormonal Balance**: The Galveston Diet emphasizes the importance of balancing hormones such as insulin, cortisol, and estrogen, which play crucial roles in metabolism and fat storage. By optimizing hormone levels through dietary and lifestyle changes, individuals can achieve and maintain a healthy weight more effectively.

2. **Anti-Inflammatory Nutrition**: Inflammation is a leading cause of various health issues, including obesity, diabetes, and heart disease. The Galveston Diet promotes anti-inflammatory foods rich in nutrients and antioxidants, such as fruits, vegetables, lean proteins, and healthy fats, while minimizing processed foods, sugars, and refined carbohydrates that contribute to inflammation.

3. **Sustainable Lifestyle Habits**: Unlike quick-fix diets that often lead to yo-yo weight fluctuations, the Galveston Diet focuses on adopting sustainable lifestyle habits that promote long-term health and well-being. This includes regular exercise, stress management techniques, adequate sleep, and mindful eating practices.

1.3   Explanation of the diet's origins and development

The Galveston Diet was developed by Dr. Mary Claire Haver, a board-certified obstetrician and gynecologist with a passion for women's health. Dr. Haver recognized the unique challenges women face when it comes to weight loss, particularly during perimenopause and menopause, when hormonal fluctuations can make it harder to maintain a healthy weight.

Drawing on her medical expertise and personal experience, Dr. Haver began researching the connections between hormones, inflammation, and weight management. She discovered that many traditional diets fail to address the underlying hormonal imbalances that contribute to stubborn weight gain, especially in women over 40.

Inspired by her findings, Dr. Haver developed the Galveston Diet as a comprehensive approach to women's health, focusing on hormonal optimization, inflammation reduction, and sustainable lifestyle changes. The diet incorporates evidence-based strategies from functional medicine, nutritional science, and behavioral psychology to provide a holistic solution for weight loss and overall wellness.

Over the years, the Galveston Diet has evolved based on ongoing research, clinical experience, and feedback from thousands of women who have successfully adopted the program. Dr. Haver continues to refine and expand the diet's offerings, including online resources, community support, and personalized coaching to help women achieve their health goals.

Lastly, the Galveston Diet offers a refreshing alternative to traditional weight loss methods, prioritizing hormonal balance, inflammation reduction, and sustainable lifestyle habits. With its evidence-based approach and focus on women's health, the Galveston Diet has the potential to empower individuals to take control of their health and transform their lives for the better.

CHAPTER TWO

2.   Understanding the Science Behind the Galveston Diet

So, let's plunge into the nitty-gritty of the Galveston Diet. But first, we need to understand the science behind it. Don't worry, I'll explain everything to you simply.

2.1   Overview of Insulin Resistance and its Role in Weight Gain

Okay, picture this: your body has this amazing hormone called insulin. Its function is to control blood sugar levels. But sometimes, your cells stop responding to insulin like they should. This is called insulin resistance, and it's a big player in weight gain.

When your cells become resistant to insulin, your body starts producing more insulin to try to compensate. This excess insulin can lead to weight gain, especially around your belly. Not cool, right?

2.2 Explanation of How the Galveston Diet Addresses Insulin Resistance

Now, here's where the Galveston Diet swoops in to save the day. This diet is all about eating in a way that keeps your blood sugar levels steady, which helps combat insulin resistance.

It focuses on wholesome, nutrient-rich foods that won't cause a big spike in your blood sugar. Think lots of veggies, lean proteins, and healthy fats. By eating this way, you can help your body better manage insulin and keep those pesky pounds at bay.

2.3 Discussion of the Hormonal Changes that Occur During Menopause and their Impact on Weight Management

Menopause; It's a time of life that many women dread, and for good reason. Along with hot flashes and mood swings, menopause can also wreak havoc on your weight.

During menopause, your hormone levels go haywire. Estrogen levels drop, which can slow down your metabolism and make it easier to pack on the pounds, especially around your midsection.

But fear not! While menopause might throw a wrench in your weight management plans, it's not game over. With the right diet and lifestyle changes, you can still keep those extra pounds in check and feel your best.

So there you have it, folks. The Galveston Diet isn't just another fad – it's backed by science and designed to help you conquer insulin resistance and navigate the hormonal ups and downs of menopause. It's time to take charge of your health and feel fabulous at any age!

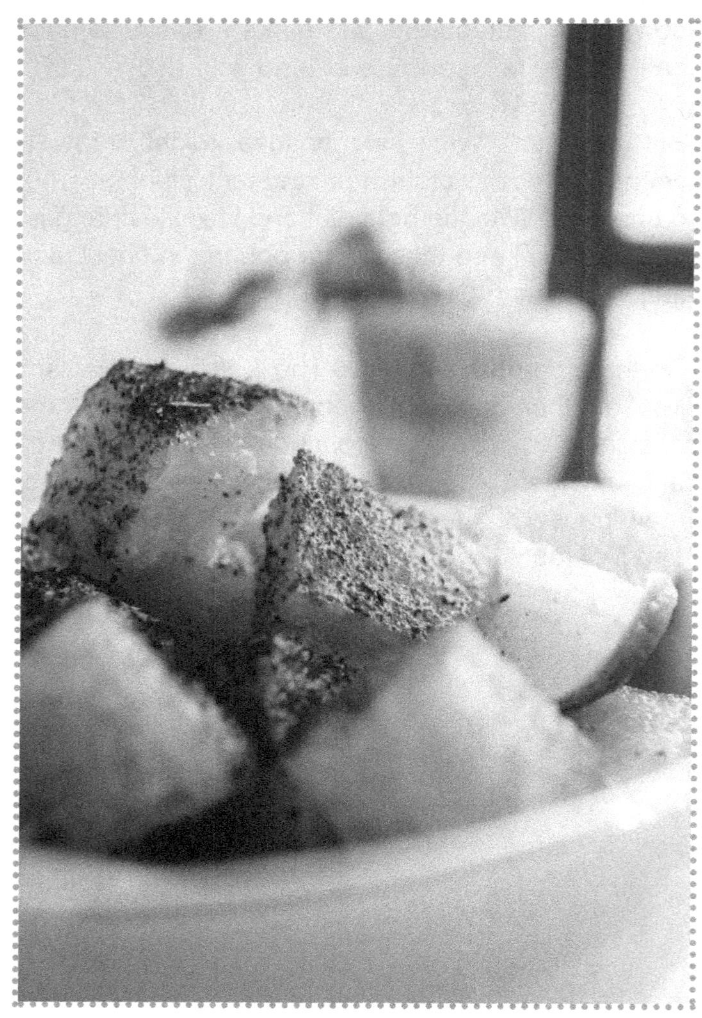

CHAPTER THREE

3. Getting Started with the Galveston Diet

So, you've decided to set out on the Galveston Diet journey? That's awesome! But before you plunge in, let's make sure you're mentally and emotionally prepared for the changes ahead.

3.1 Preparing mentally and emotionally for dietary changes

Changing your diet can be a big deal. It's not just about what you eat; it's about how you think and feel about food. Think about your motivations for wanting to make this change for a while. Maybe you want to feel healthier, have more energy, or just look better in your favorite jeans. Whatever your reasons, it's essential to be clear about them from the start.

Next, think about any challenges you might face along the way. Are there certain foods you're reluctant to give up? Do you have trouble controlling cravings or emotional eating?

By identifying potential obstacles, you can come up with strategies to overcome them.

It's also crucial to surround yourself with support. Whether it's friends, family, or an online community, having people cheering you on can make all the difference. And don't forget to be kind to yourself. Changing habits takes time, so be patient and celebrate your progress along the way.

3.2   Assessing your current dietary habits and health status

Before you can make any changes, you need to know where you're starting from. Take a close look at your current diet. On an average day, what do you eat? How often do you indulge in treats or unhealthy snacks? Be honest with yourself – this is no time for sugar-coating (pun intended).

Once you've assessed your diet, it's time to take stock of your health. Do you have any medical conditions that might affect your dietary needs? Are you taking any medications that could interact with certain foods? If you're unsure, it's always a good idea to consult with a healthcare professional.

3.3   Setting realistic goals and expectations

Now that you have a better understanding of your starting point, it's time to set some goals. But here's the key: make sure they're realistic. Sure, it would be great to drop 20 pounds in a week, but that's not going to happen (and it's not healthy either). Rather, concentrate on modest, doable objectives that you can gradually expand upon.

For example, maybe your goal is to eat more vegetables each day or cut back on sugary drinks. Or perhaps you want to cook at home more often instead of relying on takeout. Whatever your goals, make sure they're specific, measurable, and realistic.

And remember, progress is progress, no matter how small. If you slip up or don't reach your goals as quickly as you'd like, don't beat yourself up. Simply pick yourself up and continue onward. A nutritious diet and Rome weren't created in a day.

So, are you ready to get started? With the right mindset, a clear plan, and realistic goals, you're well on your way to success with the Galveston Diet. Good luck!

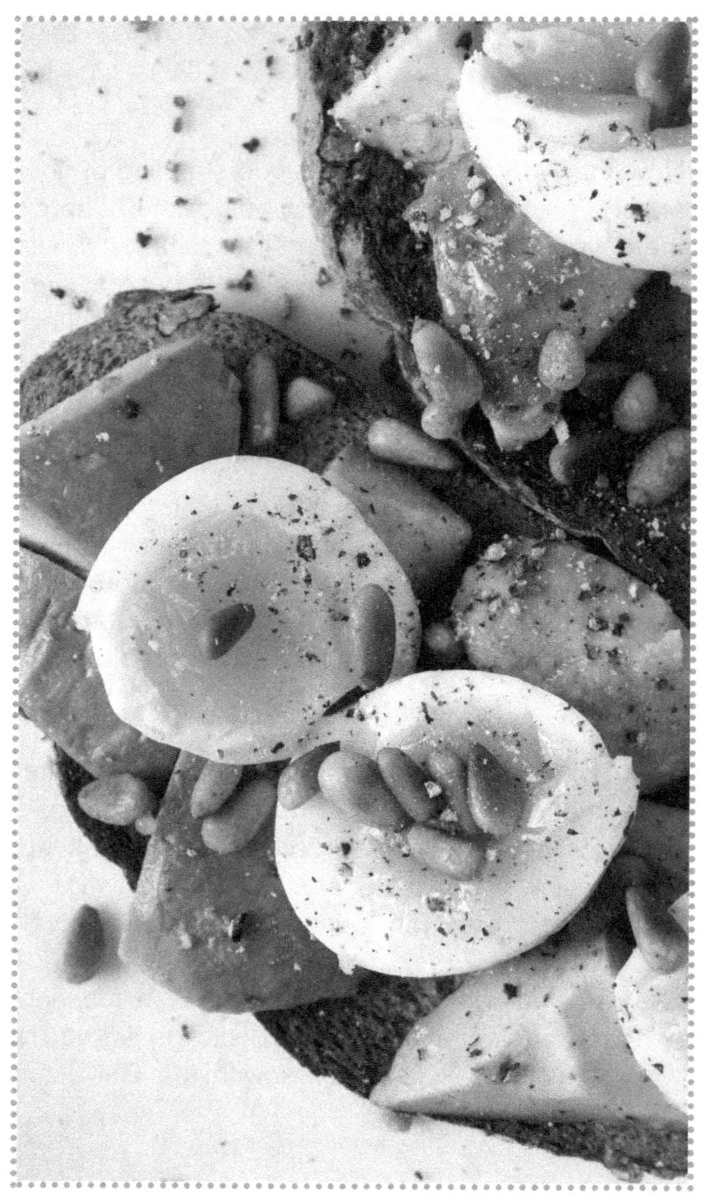

CHAPTER FOUR

4. The Galveston Diet Meal Plan

Welcome to the Galveston Diet, a comprehensive approach to nutrition designed to optimize health and promote sustainable weight loss. In this guide, we'll provide an overview of the dietary principles and guidelines, sample meal plans for different phases of the diet, and recommendations for portion sizes and meal timing to help you achieve your goals.

4.1 Overview of Dietary Principles and Guidelines

The Galveston Diet is based on the principles of balanced nutrition, blood sugar regulation, and inflammation reduction. It emphasizes whole, nutrient-dense foods while minimizing processed foods, refined sugars, and unhealthy fats. Here are some key guidelines to follow:

1. **Emphasize Protein and Healthy Fats**: Protein and healthy fats are essential for satiety, muscle repair, and hormone balance. Include sources of lean protein such as chicken, fish, eggs, and tofu, as well as healthy fats like avocados, nuts, seeds, and olive oil.

2. **Limit Carbohydrates**: While carbohydrates are not off-limits, the Galveston Diet recommends focusing on complex carbohydrates such as fruits, vegetables, and whole grains while minimizing simple carbohydrates like white bread, pasta, and sugary snacks.

3. **Eat Plenty of Vegetables**: Vegetables are rich in vitamins, minerals, and antioxidants, making them an essential part of any healthy diet. During each meal, try to have half of your plate composed of non-starchy vegetables.

4. **Manage Portion Sizes**: Pay attention to portion sizes to avoid overeating. Use smaller plates, measure your food, and practice mindful eating to tune in to your body's hunger and fullness signals.

5. **Stay Hydrated**: Drink plenty of water throughout the day to support hydration, digestion, and overall health. Limit sugary drinks and alcohol, opting for water, herbal tea, and infused water instead.

6. **Balance Blood Sugar**: Aim to eat regular meals and snacks spaced evenly throughout the day to keep blood sugar levels stable. Include protein, fiber, and healthy fats in each meal to slow

the absorption of carbohydrates and prevent spikes and crashes in blood sugar.

7. **Reduce Inflammation**: Inflammation is linked to numerous chronic diseases, so the Galveston Diet emphasizes anti-inflammatory foods such as fatty fish, leafy greens, berries, and turmeric while minimizing pro-inflammatory foods like processed meats, refined sugars, and trans fats.

4.2   Sample Meal Plans for Different Phases of the Diet

The Galveston Diet is divided into three phases: Phase 1 (Jumpstart),

Phase 2 (Balance), and

Phase 3 (Lifestyle). For each phase, here are some sample meal plans:

Phase 1: Jumpstart (2 Weeks)

During the Jumpstart phase, the focus is on kick starting weight loss and reducing inflammation.

Breakfast:

- Scrambled eggs with spinach and avocado
- Whole grain toast
- Herbal tea or black coffee

Lunch:

- Grilled chicken salad with mixed greens, tomatoes, cucumbers, and olive oil dressing
- Quinoa or brown rice

Snack:

- Greek yogurt with berries
- Handful of almonds

Dinner:

- Baked salmon with roasted vegetables (such as broccoli, carrots, and bell peppers)
- Cauliflower rice

Phase 2: Balance (Ongoing)

During the Balance phase, the focus is on maintaining weight loss and establishing healthy habits.

Breakfast:

- A smoothie with spinach, banana, almond milk, and protein powder
- Whole grain toast with almond butter

Lunch:

- Turkey and avocado wrap with whole grain tortilla
- Mixed green salad with balsamic vinaigrette

Snack:

- Hummus with carrot sticks and cucumber slices

Dinner:

- Grilled shrimp skewers with quinoa pilaf
- Steamed asparagus

Phase 3: Lifestyle (Long-Term)

During the Lifestyle phase, the focus is on sustaining healthy eating habits for the long term.

Breakfast:

- Oatmeal topped with sliced bananas, walnuts, and cinnamon
- Green tea

Lunch:

- Quinoa salad with chickpeas, cherry tomatoes, feta cheese, and lemon-tahini dressing

Snack:

- Apple slices with almond butter

Dinner:

- Grilled tofu with stir-fried vegetables (such as bell peppers, snap peas, and mushrooms)
- Brown rice

4.3   Recommendations for Portion Sizes and Meal Timing

Portion sizes and meal timing play a crucial role in the effectiveness of the Galveston Diet. Here are some recommendations:

1. **Portion Sizes**:

- Aim to fill half your plate with non-starchy vegetables, one-quarter with lean protein, and one-quarter with complex carbohydrates.

- Use your hand as a guide for portion sizes: a palm-sized portion of protein, a fist-sized portion of vegetables, a cupped hand for carbohydrates, and a thumb-sized portion of fats.

2. **Meal Timing**:

- Eat regular meals and snacks every 3-4 hours to keep blood sugar levels stable and prevent overeating.

- Avoid skipping meals, especially breakfast, as it sets the tone for the rest of the day and helps regulate appetite and energy levels.

- Pay attention to hunger and fullness cues, eating when hungry and stopping when satisfied.

By following the dietary principles and guidelines of the Galveston Diet, incorporating sample meal plans for each phase, and paying attention to portion sizes and meal timing, you can achieve your health and weight loss goals while enjoying delicious and satisfying meals. Always pay attention to your body, adjust as necessary, and acknowledge your accomplishments as you go!

CHAPTER FIVE

5.   Key Foods and Ingredients on the Galveston Diet

The Galveston Diet focuses on promoting overall health and well-being through a balance of nutritious foods. Here are some key foods and ingredients recommended on this diet:

1. **Fatty Fish**: Rich in omega-3 fatty acids, fatty fish like salmon, mackerel, and sardines are excellent sources of protein and healthy fats. These nutrients support brain function, heart health, and may even help reduce inflammation.

2. **Leafy Greens**: High in vitamins, minerals, and antioxidants are vegetables like Swiss chard, spinach, and kale. They are low in calories but high in fiber, making them ideal for supporting digestion and overall health.

3. **Berries**: Blueberries, strawberries, and raspberries are not only delicious but also loaded with antioxidants and fiber. These fruits can help protect against chronic diseases and support a healthy immune system.

4. **Nuts and Seeds**: Almonds, walnuts, chia seeds, and flaxseeds are great sources of healthy fats, protein, and fiber. They make for convenient snacks and can be added to salads, yogurt, or oatmeal for an extra nutritional boost.

5. **Healthy Fats**: Avocados, olive oil, and coconut oil are staple ingredients in the Galveston Diet. These healthy fats provide sustained energy, support brain function, and help absorb fat-soluble vitamins.

6. **Lean Protein**: Chicken breast, turkey, tofu, and legumes are excellent sources of lean protein. Protein is essential for tissue growth and repair, immune system support, and maintaining muscle mass.

7. **Whole Grains**: Quinoa, brown rice, and oats are nutritious whole grains that provide fiber, vitamins, and minerals. They help regulate blood sugar levels, support digestion, and keep you feeling full and satisfied.

5.1   Recommended Foods to Include in Your Diet

In addition to the key foods mentioned above, here are some other recommendations to include in your diet:

- **Colorful Vegetables**: Incorporate a variety of colorful vegetables like bell peppers, carrots, and tomatoes to ensure you get a wide range of nutrients.

- **Fermented Foods**: Foods like yogurt, kefir, and sauerkraut contain beneficial probiotics that support gut health and digestion.

- **Herbs and Spices**: Use herbs and spices like garlic, ginger, turmeric, and cinnamon to add flavor to your meals without extra calories or sodium.

- **Healthy Beverages**: Stay hydrated with water, herbal teas, and homemade smoothies made with fruits and vegetables.

5.2   Explanation of the Role of Macronutrients and Micronutrients

Macronutrients refer to the three main components of food that provide energy: carbohydrates, proteins, and fats.

-    **Carbohydrates**: The body uses carbohydrates as its main energy source. They are broken down into glucose, which fuels our cells and powers our brains. Carbohydrates from fruits, vegetables, whole grains, and legumes are good for you.

- **Proteins**: Building and mending tissues, producing hormones and enzymes, and bolstering the immune system all depend on proteins. Lean meats, poultry, fish, eggs, dairy products, tofu, and legumes are good sources of protein.

- **Fats**: Healthy fats are crucial for brain health, hormone production, and absorbing fat-soluble vitamins (A, D, E, and K). Olive oil, nuts, seeds, avocados, and fatty fish are good sources of healthy fats.

Micronutrients, on the other hand, are vitamins and minerals that are required in smaller quantities but are still essential for various bodily functions:

- **Vitamins**: Vitamins play vital roles in metabolism, immune function, and overall health. They include vitamin A, B vitamins, vitamin C, vitamin D, vitamin E, and vitamin K, which are found in a variety of foods like fruits, vegetables, dairy products, and fortified foods.

- **Minerals**: Minerals are essential for bone health, muscle function, fluid balance, and more. Important minerals include calcium, magnesium, potassium, sodium, iron, zinc, and selenium, which can be found in foods like leafy greens, nuts, seeds, whole grains, and lean meats.

5.3   Tips for Grocery Shopping and Meal Preparation

1. **Plan Ahead**: Take some time to plan your meals for the week and create a shopping list based on your menu. You can stay organized and refrain from impulsive purchases by doing this.

2. **Shop the Perimeter**: Focus on shopping for fresh produce, lean proteins, and dairy products around the perimeter of the grocery store. This is where you'll find the most nutritious options.

3. **Read Labels**: When purchasing packaged foods, be sure to read the nutrition labels and ingredient lists. Look for products with minimal added sugars, unhealthy fats, and artificial ingredients.

4. **Buy in Bulk**: Consider buying staple items like grains, legumes, nuts, and seeds in bulk to save money and reduce packaging waste.

5. **Meal Prep**: Dedicate some time each week to meal prep by chopping vegetables, cooking grains, and pre-portioning snacks. This will make it easier to assemble healthy meals throughout the week, especially on busy days.

6. **Experiment with Recipes**: Don't be afraid to try new recipes and experiment with different flavors and ingredients. Cooking at home allows you to control the quality of your meals and tailor them to your taste preferences.

7. **Stay Flexible**: Remember that it's okay to be flexible with your meal plan and make substitutions based on what's available or in season. Focus on incorporating a variety of nutrient-dense foods into your diet for optimal health.

By following these tips and incorporating key foods and ingredients into your diet, you can support your overall health and well-being on the Galveston Diet.

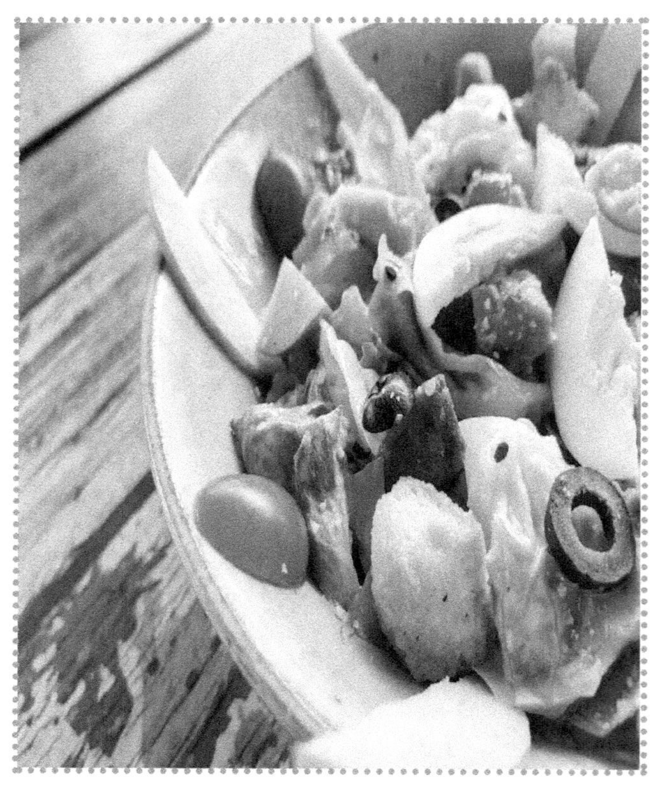

CHAPTER SIX

6.   Incorporating Exercise and Physical Activity

Physical activity and exercise are crucial elements of a healthy lifestyle. They not only contribute to weight management but also promote overall well-being. Incorporating exercise into your daily routine can seem daunting at first, but with the right approach, it can become an enjoyable and rewarding habit.

6.2   Importance of Regular Physical Activity for Overall Health and Weight Management

Regular physical activity offers numerous benefits for both your body and mind. It helps to improve cardiovascular health, strengthen muscles and bones, and boost immune function. Additionally, exercise plays a crucial role in weight management by burning calories and increasing metabolism.

Engaging in regular physical activity can also reduce the risk of chronic diseases such as heart disease, diabetes, and certain types of cancer.

Furthermore, exercise has been shown to improve mood and mental health by reducing symptoms of anxiety and depression.

6.3 Types of Exercise Recommended on the Galveston Diet

The Galveston Diet emphasizes a combination of aerobic exercise, strength training, and flexibility exercises to support weight loss and overall health. Aerobic exercise, such as walking, jogging, or cycling, helps to burn calories and improve cardiovascular fitness.

Strength training, which involves using resistance to build muscle strength and endurance, is also an important component of the Galveston Diet. This can include exercises like weight lifting, bodyweight exercises, or using resistance bands.

In addition to aerobic and strength training, flexibility exercises such as yoga or stretching are recommended to improve joint mobility and reduce the risk of injury.

6.4   Strategies   for   Incorporating Exercise into Your Daily Routine

It is not difficult to incorporate exercise into your daily routine. With some planning and creativity, you can find ways to stay active throughout the day. The strategies listed below will help you get going:

1. **Schedule It:** Treat exercise like any other appointment and schedule it into your day. Whether it's a morning walk, a lunchtime yoga class, or an evening gym session, setting aside dedicated time for exercise can help ensure you prioritize it.

2.**Find Activities You Enjoy:** Try out various forms of physical activity until you discover things that you actually look forward to doing. Whether it's dancing, swimming, or hiking, choosing activities that you look forward to makes it easier to stick with them long term.

3. **Make It Social:** Exercise doesn't have to be a solo activity. Invite friends or family members to join you for a workout or participate in group fitness classes. Not only does this make exercise more enjoyable, but it also provides accountability and support.

4. **Incorporate Movement Throughout the Day:** Look for opportunities to incorporate movement into your daily routine. Take the stairs instead of the elevator, walk or bike to work if possible, or do bodyweight exercises while watching TV. Every little bit of movement adds up!

5. **Set Realistic Goals:** Set achievable goals for your exercise routine, whether it's completing a certain number of workouts per week or increasing your daily step count. Start small and gradually increase the intensity or duration of your workouts as you progress.

6. **Track Your Progress:** Keep track of your exercise habits and progress towards your goals. This could be through a fitness app, a journal, or simply marking your workouts on a calendar. You can stay motivated and on track by keeping an eye on your progress.

7. **Be Flexible:** Life can be unpredictable, and there will be times when sticking to a rigid exercise schedule is challenging. Be adaptable and ready to change your routine when necessary. Keep in mind that movement of any kind is preferable to none at all.

By incorporating exercise into your daily routine and making it a priority, you can reap the numerous benefits it offers for both your physical and mental health. Whether it's a brisk walk in the park, a yoga class with friends, or a solo strength training session at the gym, find what works best for you and make it a regular part of your life. You'll feel the benefits in your body and mind!

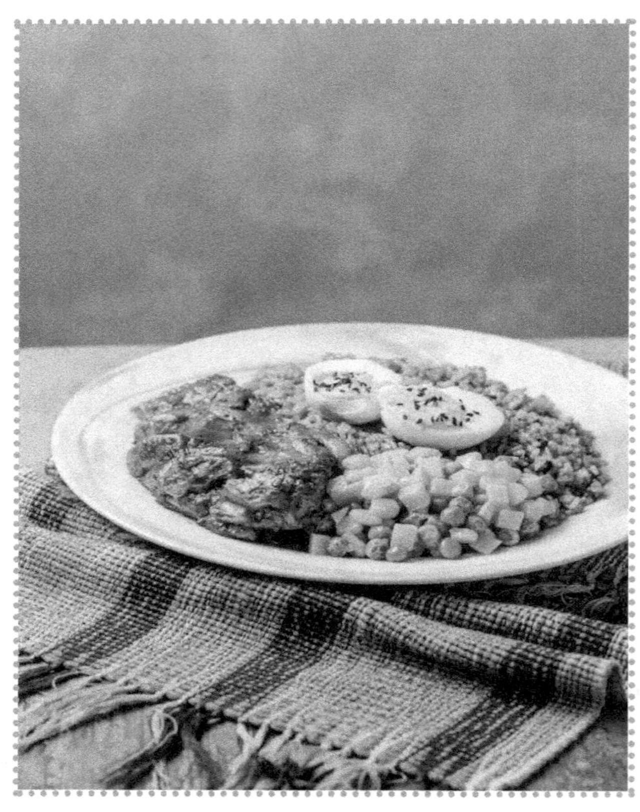

CHAPTER SEVEN

7. Steering Challenges and Overcoming Plateaus

When it comes to following any diet, bumps in the road are almost inevitable. The Galveston Diet, like any other plan, has its own set of challenges and plateaus that can make the journey feel like a rollercoaster ride. But fear not! With the right strategies and mindset, you can overcome these obstacles and keep moving forward towards your health goals.

7.2 Common obstacles encountered while following the Galveston Diet

One of the most common hurdles people face on the Galveston Diet is adjusting to the new way of eating. Saying goodbye to certain foods you love and embracing healthier alternatives can be tough at first. It's natural to experience cravings and feelings of deprivation, especially in the beginning. Additionally, life's unpredictable nature can throw curveballs your way, making it challenging to stick to your diet plan.

There are a lot of things that can stop you from making progress, like parties, hectic schedules, or stress eating.

7.3. Strategies for overcoming cravings and maintaining motivation

Cravings are like little roadblocks on your journey to better health, but they don't have to stop you in your tracks. One effective strategy is to be prepared with healthy alternatives to your favorite treats. Stock your pantry and fridge with nutritious snacks like fruits, nuts, and veggies to satisfy cravings without derailing your diet. Additionally, practicing mindfulness and tuning in to your body's hunger cues can help you distinguish between true hunger and emotional cravings.

Another key to staying motivated is finding your "why." Remind yourself of the reasons you started this journey in the first place. Whether it's improving your health, boosting your energy levels, or feeling more confident in your own skin, keeping your goals front and center can help you stay focused when temptation strikes. Surround yourself with a supportive community, whether it's friends, family, or online groups, who can cheer you on during the tough times and celebrate your victories along the way.

7.4 Tips for breaking through weight loss plateaus

Plateaus are frustrating, but they're also a natural part of the weight loss journey. When your body gets used to your new eating habits and activity level, it can sometimes hit a standstill, making it difficult to shed those last few pounds. But don't despair! There are several strategies you can try to kick-start your progress again.

First, shake things up with your exercise routine. Your body may have adapted to your current workouts, so try adding new activities or increasing the intensity to challenge yourself in different ways. Similarly, mixing up your diet can help jumpstart your metabolism and reignite weight loss. Experiment with new recipes, incorporate more variety into your meals, and pay attention to portion sizes to ensure you're not overeating.

Additionally, don't forget the importance of sleep and stress management in your weight loss journey. Lack of sleep and high stress levels can wreak havoc on your hormones, making it harder to lose weight. Prioritize self-care and relaxation techniques like meditation, yoga, or deep breathing exercises to keep your mind and body in balance.

Ultimately, while steering the challenges and plateaus of the Galveston Diet may seem daunting at times, with the right strategies and mindset, you can overcome any obstacle that comes your way. Stay focused on your goals, surround yourself with support, and remember that every step forward, no matter how small, brings you closer to a healthier, happier you.

CHAPTER EIGHT

8. Monitoring Progress and Adjusting Your Approach

When it comes to reaching your health and fitness goals, monitoring your progress is key. It's like navigating a ship; you need to keep checking your compass to ensure you're headed in the right direction. But it's not just about checking off boxes; it's about understanding where you are, where you want to be, and how to adjust your course if needed.

8.2 Importance of Tracking Your Food Intake, Exercise, and Progress

Think of tracking your food intake and exercise as keeping a diary of your journey. It's not just about calories in versus calories out; it's about understanding what you're putting into your body and how it affects your overall health. By tracking your food intake, you can identify patterns, pinpoint areas for improvement, and make informed decisions about your diet.

Likewise, tracking your exercise allows you to see how active you've been and if you're meeting your fitness goals. It's not just about hitting the gym for an hour and calling it a day; it's about consistent effort and progress over time.

And of course, tracking your progress is essential for staying motivated and focused. Whether it's recording your weight, body measurements, or even how you feel mentally and emotionally, keeping track allows you to celebrate your successes and identify areas where you can improve.

8.3 How to Interpret Changes in Weight and Body Measurements

One of the most common ways people track their progress is by stepping on the scale. But weight alone doesn't tell the whole story. It's important to understand that your weight can fluctuate for various reasons, including water retention, muscle gain, and even the time of day you weigh yourself.

Instead of focusing solely on the number on the scale, pay attention to how your clothes fit and how you feel in your body. Body measurements, such as waist circumference and body fat percentage, can also provide valuable insights into your progress.

For example, if you notice that your clothes are fitting looser and your waist measurement is decreasing, even if the scale hasn't budged, it could mean that you're losing fat and developing muscle, which is a good development.

On the other hand, if you're consistently gaining weight or your body measurements are increasing, it could indicate that you need to reassess your diet and exercise routine.

8.4 Making Adjustments to Your Diet and Exercise Routine as Needed

Once you've been tracking your food intake, exercise, and progress for a while, you may start to notice patterns and trends. Maybe you've hit a plateau in your weight loss journey, or perhaps you're not seeing the muscle gains you'd hoped for.

This is where making adjustments to your diet and exercise routine comes in. Instead of getting discouraged, use this information to refine your approach and keep moving forward.

For example, if you've hit a plateau in your weight loss, try adjusting your calorie intake or incorporating more high-intensity workouts into your routine. If you're not seeing the muscle gains you want, consider increasing your protein intake and focusing on strength training exercises.

It's important to approach these adjustments with patience and consistency. A healthy body takes time to develop, just like Rome wasn't built in a day. By continually monitoring your progress and making small tweaks along the way, you can stay on track to reaching your health and fitness goals.

Lastly, monitoring your progress and adjusting your approach is essential for achieving success in your health and fitness journey. By tracking your food intake, exercise, and progress, interpreting changes in weight and body measurements, and making adjustments to your diet and exercise routine as needed, you can stay committed, driven, and on course to accomplish your objectives . Remember, it's not about perfection; it's about progress. Keep pushing forward, and you'll get there.

CHAPTER NINE

9. Sustaining-Long-Term Success with the Galveston Diet

The Galveston Diet is a lifestyle approach to eating that focuses on nourishing your body with wholesome foods while promoting overall health and well-being. But sustaining long-term success with any diet requires more than just following a set of guidelines; it involves adopting sustainable habits and making mindful choices every day.

9.2 Strategies for maintaining weight loss and healthy habits

Once you've achieved your desired weight loss with the Galveston Diet, the challenge becomes keeping the weight off and staying healthy in the long run. Here are some effective strategies to help you maintain your progress:

1. **Stay Consistent:** Consistency is key to long-term success. Stick to the principles of the Galveston Diet even after reaching your goal weight. This means continuing to prioritize whole, nutrient-rich foods while limiting processed and sugary treats.

2. **Find Balance:** The Galveston Diet emphasizes a balance of macronutrients, including healthy fats, lean proteins, and complex carbohydrates. Maintaining this balance can help you fuel your body properly and keep cravings in check.

3. **Incorporate Exercise:** Regular physical activity is essential for maintaining weight loss and overall health. Include exercise on a regular basis in your routine and engage in activities you enjoy. Whether it's walking, swimming, or cycling, find what works for you and stick with it.

4. **Practice Mindful Eating:** Pay attention to your hunger and fullness cues, and eat slowly to savor your food. Avoid distractions while eating, such as watching TV or scrolling through your phone, as this can lead to overeating.

5. **Monitor Your Progress:** Keep track of your food intake, exercise routine, and progress toward your goals. This can help you stay accountable and make adjustments as needed to maintain your weight loss.

9.3 Tips for dining out and social occasions while following the Galveston Diet

Eating out and attending social events can present challenges when following any diet, including the Galveston Diet. However, with some planning and preparation, you can navigate these situations while staying true to your health goals. Here are some tips:

1. **Plan Ahead:** Before dining out, take a look at the menu online and choose options that align with the principles of the Galveston Diet. Look for dishes that are rich in lean proteins, healthy fats, and vegetables, and ask for dressings and sauces on the side.

2. **Be Mindful of Portions:** Restaurant portions are often larger than what you would typically eat at home. Consider sharing an entree with a friend or asking for a to-go box to save half for later.

3. **Make Smart Substitutions:** Don't be afraid to ask for substitutions or modifications to make a dish more Galveston Diet-friendly. For example, request grilled or steamed vegetables instead of fries, or a side salad instead of a starchy side dish.

4. **Watch Your Beverages:** Be mindful of what you're drinking, as beverages can contribute a significant amount of calories and sugar to your meal. Opt for water, unsweetened tea, or sparkling water with lemon or lime instead of sugary sodas or alcoholic beverages.

5. **Focus on Enjoyment:** Remember that dining out is also about enjoying the experience and socializing with friends and family. Focus on the company and conversation rather than just the food.

9.4 Incorporating flexibility and balance into your lifestyle

While following the Galveston Diet can provide structure and guidance for making healthy choices, it's essential to also incorporate flexibility and balance into your lifestyle. Here are some ways to do that:

1. **Allow for Treats:** It's okay to indulge in your favorite treats occasionally. The key is moderation and mindfulness. Enjoy a small portion of your favorite dessert or snack without guilt, and then return to your regular healthy eating habits.

2. **Practice Self-Compassion:** Be kind to yourself and recognize that perfection is not

attainable. If you veer off track occasionally, don't beat yourself up. Instead, focus on making the next choice a healthy one and move forward.

3. **Find Activities You Enjoy:** In addition to exercise, find other activities that bring you joy and help reduce stress. Whether it's yoga, meditation, gardening, or spending time with loved ones, prioritize activities that nourish your mind, body, and soul.

4. **Listen to Your Body:** Take note of your body's reactions to various foods and modify your diet accordingly. If certain foods leave you feeling sluggish or bloated, consider reducing or eliminating them from your diet.

5. **Be Flexible:** Life is unpredictable, and there will be times when sticking to a strict diet plan is challenging. Instead of viewing these situations as setbacks, see them as opportunities to practice flexibility and resilience. Make the best choices you can with the options available to you, and trust that you can get back on track when things settle down.

Finally, sustaining long-term success with the Galveston Diet requires commitment, consistency, and flexibility. By following these strategies and tips, you can maintain your weight loss, support your overall health, and enjoy a balanced and fulfilling lifestyle for years to come.

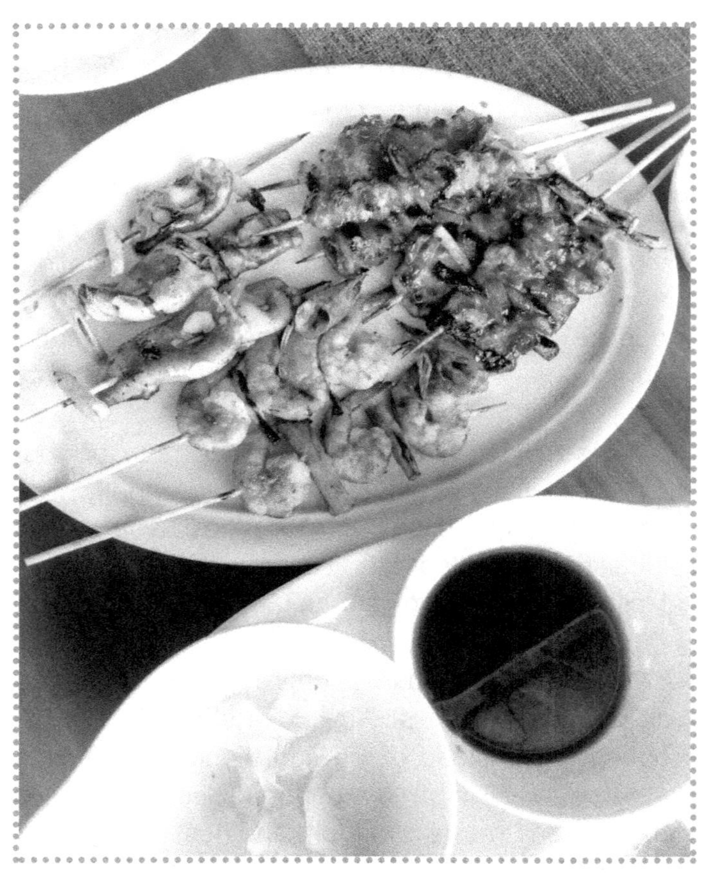

CHAPTER TEN

10.   Additional Resources and Support

Looking for more information and assistance with the Galveston Diet? You're in the right place! Whether you're seeking further reading materials, online communities, or professional guidance, we've got you covered. Let's dive into the resources available to support your journey.

10.2   Recommended Books, and Other Resources for Further Reading

- **Books**:

1. ***"The Galveston Diet**: Unlocking the Secret to Lifelong Health"** by Dr. Mary Claire Haver - This book is the ultimate guide to understanding the Galveston Diet, written by its creator. Dr. Haver provides in-depth explanations, meal plans, and recipes to help you implement the diet successfully.

2. ***"The Hormone Reset Die**t"** by Dr. Sara Gottfried - While not specifically about the Galveston Diet, this book delves into the importance of hormone balance for overall health,

which aligns with the principles of the Galveston approach.

- **Other Resources**:

1. **Podcasts and Webinars** - Look for podcasts or webinars featuring Dr. Mary Claire Haver or other experts discussing topics related to women's health, intermittent fasting, and hormonal balance.

2. **Nutrition Apps** - Consider using nutrition tracking apps like MyFitnessPal or Cronometer to help you stay on track with your dietary goals and monitor your progress.

10.3   Information on Joining Online Communities   or   Support   Groups Related to the Galveston Diet

Connecting with others who are following the Galveston Diet can provide invaluable support, motivation, and insights. Here are some ways to join online communities or support groups:

1. **Facebook Groups** - Search for Facebook groups dedicated to the Galveston Diet or related topics such as intermittent fasting, women's health, or hormone optimization. These groups often serve as forums for sharing experiences, asking questions, and offering support.

2. **Reddit Communities** - Explore subreddits like r/GalvestonDiet or r/IntermittentFasting to engage with others who are on a similar journey. Reddit can be a great place to find community support and access to a wealth of knowledge and experiences.

3. **Online Forums** - Look for forums or message boards hosted on health and wellness websites where members discuss the Galveston Diet and related topics. Websites like Bodybuilding.com or Healthline may have active communities focused on intermittent fasting and women's health.

4. **Instagram and Twitter** - Follow hashtags related to the Galveston Diet on social media platforms like Instagram and Twitter to connect with like-minded individuals, share your progress, and discover tips and inspiration from others.

10.4 Options for Seeking Professional Guidance or Coaching Support

If you're looking for personalized guidance or additional support on your Galveston Diet journey, consider the following options:

1. **Certified Galveston Diet Coaches** - The Galveston Diet website offers access to certified coaches who can provide personalized guidance, support, and accountability to help you achieve your health goals. These coaches are trained in the principles of the Galveston approach and can tailor their support to your individual needs.

2. **Nutritionists or Dietitians** - Consider working with a registered dietitian or nutritionist who can provide evidence-based guidance on implementing the Galveston Diet in a way that

meets your unique dietary preferences, health concerns, and lifestyle.

3. **Health Coaches** - Health coaches specialize in helping clients make sustainable lifestyle changes to improve their overall health and well-being. Look for a health coach who is familiar with the principles of the Galveston Diet and can provide holistic support in areas such as nutrition, exercise, stress management, and sleep.

4. **Online Programs and Courses** - Explore online programs or courses offered by reputable health and wellness professionals that focus on the principles of the Galveston Diet. These programs may include educational materials, meal plans, coaching support, and community forums to help you succeed.

By utilizing these additional resources, joining supportive communities, and seeking professional guidance, you can enhance your experience with the Galveston Diet and optimize your journey toward better health and well-being. Remember, every step you take toward prioritizing your health is a step in the right direction!

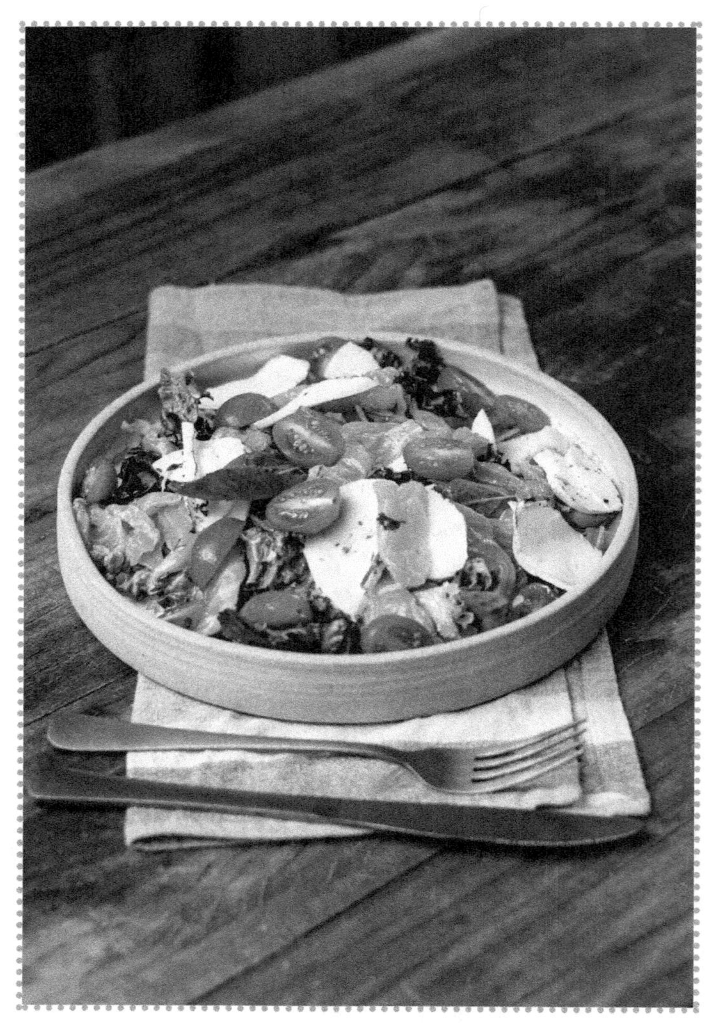

CHAPTER ELEVEN

11. FAQs and Common Concerns about the Galveston Diet

Are you considering trying out the Galveston Diet? Maybe you've heard about it from a friend or stumbled upon it online. Whatever the case, it's natural to have questions and concerns before embarking on any new diet plan. In this comprehensive guide, we'll address the most frequently asked questions about the Galveston Diet and dispel any common concerns or misconceptions you might have.

1. What is the Galveston Diet?

The Galveston Diet is a nutrition plan designed specifically for women who are experiencing hormonal changes, particularly during perimenopause and menopause. Created by Dr. Mary Claire Haver, an OB-GYN with a passion for women's health, this diet aims to optimize hormone balance and promote weight loss through targeted dietary changes.

2. How does the Galveston Diet work?

The Galveston Diet works by focusing on the types of foods that can support hormone balance and metabolic function in women. It emphasizes whole foods, healthy fats, lean proteins, and low-glycemic carbohydrates while minimizing processed foods, sugars, and refined grains. By following this approach, women may experience improved energy levels, better mood stability, and weight loss.

3. Is the Galveston Diet safe?

Yes, the Galveston Diet is generally safe for most women, particularly those experiencing symptoms of hormonal imbalance. However, as with any diet or lifestyle change, it's essential to consult with a healthcare provider before starting, especially if you have any underlying health conditions or concerns.

4. Will I lose weight on the Galveston Diet?

Weight loss can be a common outcome of following the Galveston Diet, especially for women who are experiencing hormonal fluctuations that may contribute to weight gain. However, individual results may vary, and factors such as adherence to the diet, activity level, and metabolism can influence weight loss success.

5. Are there any side effects of the Galveston Diet?

While the Galveston Diet is designed to promote overall health and well-being, some women may experience temporary side effects, especially during the initial phase of dietary change. These side effects can include mild digestive discomfort, changes in energy levels, or fluctuations in mood. However, these symptoms typically subside as the body adjusts to the new eating plan.

6. Can I follow the Galveston Diet if I have dietary restrictions?

The Galveston Diet can be adapted to accommodate various dietary restrictions, including gluten-free, dairy-free, or vegetarian preferences. With its focus on whole, nutrient-dense foods, there is plenty of flexibility to customize the diet to meet individual needs while still supporting hormone balance and weight loss goals.

7. How long should I follow the Galveston Diet?

The length of time you follow the Galveston Diet may depend on your individual goals and health status. Some women may choose to follow the plan for a specific period, such as several weeks or months, to kickstart weight loss or address hormonal symptoms. Others may adopt it as a long-term lifestyle approach for ongoing health and wellness.

11.2 Common Concerns and Misconceptions

Now that we've covered some frequently asked questions about the Galveston Diet, let's address some common concerns and misconceptions that you might have encountered.

1. **Concern**: The Galveston Diet is too restrictive.

Some people may worry that the Galveston Diet is too restrictive, particularly if they enjoy a wide variety of foods or have specific dietary preferences. However, while the diet does emphasize certain food groups over others, it's designed to be flexible and sustainable for long-term adherence. With a focus on whole, nutrient-dense foods, there is still plenty of room for creativity and enjoyment in meal planning.

2. **Concern**: I won't get enough nutrients on the Galveston Diet.

Another concern that some people may have is whether they'll get enough essential nutrients while following the Galveston Diet. However, the diet is carefully crafted to provide a balance of macronutrients (such as carbohydrates, proteins, and fats) and micronutrients (such as vitamins and minerals) necessary for overall health and well-being. By prioritizing whole foods and minimizing processed items, the Galveston Diet can actually enhance nutrient intake compared to a typical Western diet.

3. **Concern**: The Galveston Diet won't work for me.

It's understandable to feel skeptical about trying a new diet plan, especially if you've tried others in the past without success. However, the Galveston Diet is specifically tailored to address the unique hormonal challenges that women face, particularly during perimenopause and menopause. By targeting hormone balance through dietary changes, many women have experienced positive outcomes such as weight loss, increased energy, and improved mood.

4. **Concern**: I'll miss my favorite foods on the Galveston Diet.

Transitioning to any new diet plan can be challenging, especially if it requires giving up certain foods that you enjoy. However, the Galveston Diet encourages a balanced approach to eating that allows for occasional treats and indulgences in moderation. By focusing on nourishing your body with whole, nutrient-dense foods most of the time, you can still enjoy your favorite treats occasionally without derailing your progress.

5. **Concern**: The Galveston Diet is too expensive.

Some people may worry that following the Galveston Diet will be too expensive, particularly if it requires purchasing specialty or organic foods. While it's true that some healthier food options may come with a higher price tag, there are plenty of budget-friendly ways to follow the Galveston Diet. By prioritizing whole foods, buying in bulk, and planning meals ahead of time, you can make the most of your grocery budget while still nourishing your body with quality ingredients.

Finally, the Galveston Diet offers a tailored approach to nutrition that can support hormone balance, promote weight loss, and enhance overall health and well-being for women experiencing perimenopause and menopause. By addressing common concerns and misconceptions, we hope to provide clarity and guidance for those considering this dietary approach. As always, it's essential to consult with a healthcare provider before making any significant changes to your diet or lifestyle to ensure that it aligns with your individual needs and goals.

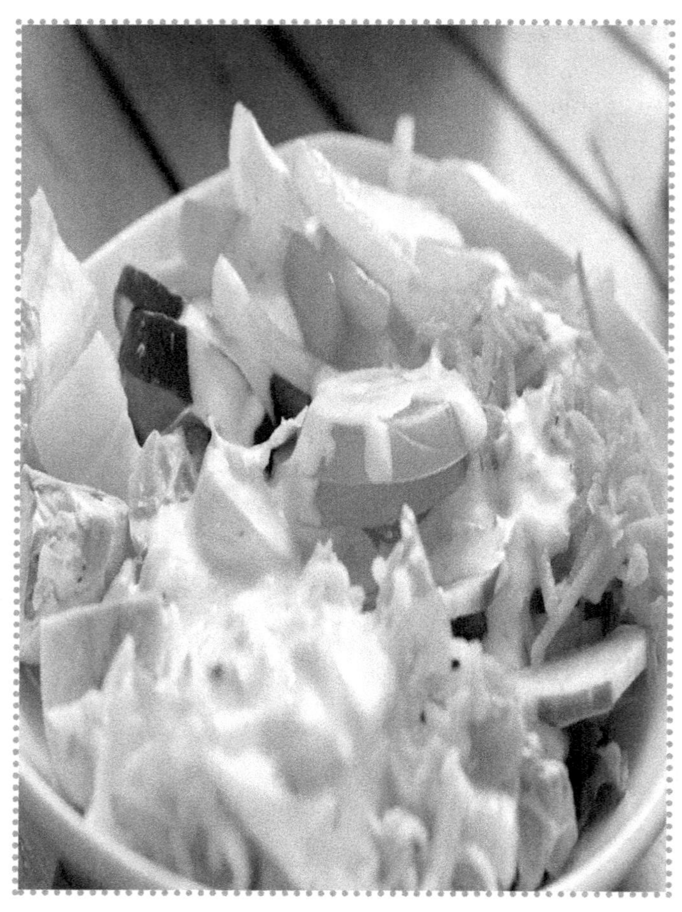

CHAPTER TWELVE

12. Conclusion:

Congratulations on completing your journey through the Galveston Diet! As you reflect on the principles and takeaways, it's essential to celebrate your achievements and acknowledge the progress you've made towards better health and well-being. Remember, this isn't just about reaching a certain weight or fitting into a specific size; it's about cultivating sustainable habits that support your overall vitality and longevity.

12.2 Recap of Key Principles:

The Galveston Diet is more than just a meal plan; it's a holistic approach to health that emphasizes nourishing your body with nutrient-dense foods, balancing hormones, and reducing inflammation. Here's a recap of some key principles you've learned along the way:

1. **Balancing Hormones**: By focusing on foods that support hormonal balance, such as healthy fats, lean proteins, and fiber-rich

carbohydrates, you've been able to regulate insulin levels, curb cravings, and optimize metabolism.

2. **Reducing Inflammation**: Inflammation is a root cause of many chronic diseases, including obesity, diabetes, and heart disease. Through the Galveston Diet, you've learned to prioritize anti-inflammatory foods like fatty fish, leafy greens, berries, and nuts, while minimizing pro-inflammatory foods like refined sugars and processed foods.

3. **Intermittent Fasting**: Intermittent fasting has been a cornerstone of your journey, helping to improve insulin sensitivity, promote fat loss, and enhance cellular repair and regeneration. By incorporating fasting periods into your routine, you've tapped into your body's natural ability to heal and rejuvenate.

4. **Mindful Eating**: Eating mindfully involves paying attention to hunger and fullness cues, savoring each bite, and being present during meals. This practice not only fosters a healthier relationship with food but also helps prevent overeating and promote digestion.

5. **Lifestyle Factors**: Beyond nutrition, the Galveston Diet emphasizes the importance of lifestyle factors such as regular physical activity, adequate sleep, stress management, and social support. These elements are essential for overall well-being and complement the dietary principles of the program.

12.3 Takeaways:

As you move forward on your health journey, here are some key takeaways to keep in mind:

1. **Consistency is Key**: Sustainable change takes time and consistency. Continue to prioritize healthy eating habits, regular exercise, and self-care practices, even when faced with challenges or setbacks.

2. **Listen to Your Body**: Your body is incredibly wise and will often communicate its needs and preferences. Observe your reactions to various foods and modify your diet accordingly. Remember, there's no one-size-fits-all approach to nutrition, so trust your instincts and intuition.

3. **Embrace Variety**: Keep your meals interesting and diverse by experimenting with new ingredients, flavors, and cuisines. Eating a wide range of foods not only ensures you're getting a

variety of nutrients but also prevents boredom and monotony.

4. **Stay Mindful**: Continue practicing mindful eating by tuning into your body's hunger and fullness signals, as well as the sensory experience of eating. Avoid distractions like screens or multitasking during meals, and savor each bite with gratitude and awareness.

5. **Celebrate Progress**: Celebrate your victories, no matter how small. Whether it's fitting into a pair of jeans you haven't worn in years or noticing improvements in energy levels and mood, take time to acknowledge and celebrate your progress along the way.

12.4 Encouragement for Continued Success:

As you continue your journey towards optimal health and vitality, remember that you're not alone. Surround yourself with a supportive community of like-minded individuals who share similar goals and values. Lean on friends, family, or online support groups for encouragement, accountability, and inspiration.

Be patient and compassionate with yourself, recognizing that change is a gradual process, and setbacks are a natural part of the journey. Instead of dwelling on past mistakes or perceived failures, focus on what you can control in the present moment and commit to making positive choices moving forward.

Above all, prioritize self-care and self-love in all aspects of your life. Treat yourself with kindness, respect, and compassion, honoring your body, mind, and spirit. Remember that true health and happiness come from within and are not defined by external measures or societal standards.

By embracing the principles of the Galveston Diet and integrating them into your daily life with intention and mindfulness, you're not only transforming your physical health but also nurturing a deeper sense of well-being and vitality. Trust in the process, believe in yourself, and know that you have everything you need to succeed on this incredible journey towards lasting health and happiness.

12.5. DAILY MEAL REMAKE

S/N	DAILY	MEAL	REMAKE